MW01247555

The Complete Guide to Fasting

Log, Journal and Workbook

The Complete Guide to Fasting Log, Journal and Workbook
Based on Dr. Jason Fung's Principles for Fasting for Health
and Weight Loss

Copyright © 2019, ItsAboutTimeBooks.com
All rights reserved.

No parts of this publication may be reproduced, stored in a
retrieval system, or transmitted in any form or by any
means, electronic, mechanical, photocopying, recording, or
otherwise, without the prior written permission of the
copyright owner.

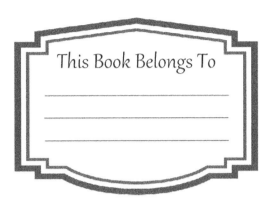

This Book Belongs To

_____

_____

_____

How to Use This Book

The Complete Guide to Fasting Log, Journal and Workbook covers a 6-month period includes the following ages:

CALENDAR: A blank month-at-glance calendar for you to plug in the dates of the current month along with any details – holidays, work schedules, planned or actual fasts, etc. Whatever you think is appropriate or needed.

GOALS and INTENTIONS: A page where you can enter weekly goals or intentions. You could use this to jot down your planned fasting schedule, your weight-loss and/or exercise goals, etc. You can also use it for purely personal or business goals and intentions.

WEEKLY PLANNER PAGE: 5 blank weekly calendar/planner pages per month on the left-hand side to use as you would a regular planner – appointments, to do lists, etc. (or however you like).

WEEKLY JOURNAL TRACKER PAGES: 5 corresponding weekly journal / tracker pages on the right-hand page. Use these for jotting down your foods or other notes -- plus a grid where you can enter Start and End times for any fasts you're doing, your macro counts (calories, carbs, fat, and protein) for the day, and whether or not you have a journal entry for the day.

REFLECTION PAGES: Two pages where you can answer the questions, *Did I fulfill my intentions (goals) for the month? What went right? What went wrong?* And on the second Reflection page, *What steps can I take to improve my results next month? Biggest lesson learned,? Reward for the month?* And finally, *NSVs* (Non-Scale Victories) for the month such as close fitting looser, lower A1C readings, symptoms clearing up, etc.

MISCELLANEOUS NOTES: Two pages to journal any thoughts, experience, etc. during the month – and for which you checked the Journal entry block in your tracker grid. You might want to record great menus, recipe ideas, symptoms you've had (or lost!), fasting experience, emotions, etc. And there are 10 more notes pages at the back of the book.

In short: everything you need to plan and execute your fasting regimen.

Please share any comments, suggestions or ideas with us:
Info@ItsAboutTimeBooks.com

And don't forget to leave a review!

Measurements

	Start	Month 1	Month 2	Month 3
Bust	Date	Date	Date	Date
Waist				
Hips				
Arms				
Thigh				
Calf				
Weight				

Additional Notes:

Measurements

	Month 4	Month 5	Month 6
Bust	Date	Date	Date
Waist			
Hips			
Arms			
Thigh			
Calf			
Weight			

Additional Notes:

Month _____ *Year* _____

SUN	MON	TUES	WED	THURS	FRI	SAT

GOALS AND INTENTIONS FOR THE MONTH

Week 1

1. _____

2. _____

3. _____

_____

Week 2

1. _____

2. _____

3. _____

_____

Week 3

1. _____

2. _____

3. _____

_____

Week 4

1. _____

2. _____

3. _____

_____

Month 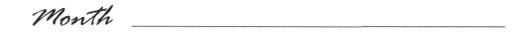 _____

SUNDAY
_____

GOALS/ PRIORITIES
_____
_____
_____
_____

MONDAY
_____
_____
_____
_____
_____

TUESDAY
_____
_____
_____
_____
_____
_____

WEDNESDAY
_____
_____

TASKS / TO DOs
_____
_____
_____

THURSDAY
_____
_____
_____
_____

FRIDAY
_____
_____
_____
_____

SATURDAY
_____
_____

Month 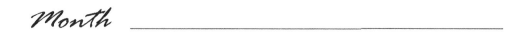 _____

SUNDAY _____

GOALS/ PRIORITIES _____

_____

_____

_____

_____

MONDAY _____

_____

_____

_____

_____

TUESDAY _____

_____

_____

_____

_____

WEDNESDAY _____

_____

TASKS / TO DOs _____

_____

_____

THURSDAY _____

_____

_____

_____

_____

FRIDAY _____

_____

_____

_____

_____

SATURDAY _____

_____

_____

Month _____

	Start Fast	End Fast	Calories	Carbs	Fat	Protein	Journal?
SUNDAY							
MONDAY							
TUESDAY							
WEDNESDAY							
THURSDAY							
FRIDAY							
SATURDAY							

Month 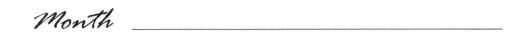 _____

SUNDAY _____

GOALS/ PRIORITIES

_____

_____

_____

_____

MONDAY _____

_____

_____

_____

_____

_____

_____

TUESDAY _____

_____

_____

_____

_____

_____

WEDNESDAY _____

_____

TASKS / TO DOs

_____

_____

_____

THURSDAY _____

_____

_____

_____

_____

_____

FRIDAY _____

_____

_____

_____

_____

_____

SATURDAY _____

_____

_____

Month _____

	Start Fast	End Fast	Calories	Carbs	Fat	Protein	Journal?
SUNDAY							
MONDAY							
TUESDAY							
WEDNESDAY							
THURSDAY							
FRIDAY							
SATURDAY							

Month _____

	Start Fast	End Fast	Calories	Carbs	Fat	Protein	Journal?
SUNDAY							
MONDAY							
TUESDAY							
WEDNESDAY							
THURSDAY							
FRIDAY							
SATURDAY							

Month 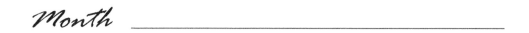 _____

SUNDAY
_____

MONDAY
_____

TUESDAY
_____

WEDNESDAY
_____

THURSDAY
_____

FRIDAY
_____

SATURDAY
_____

GOALS/ PRIORITIES
_____
_____
_____
_____
_____
_____
_____
_____
_____
_____
_____
_____
_____
_____

TASKS / TO DOs
_____
_____
_____
_____
_____
_____
_____
_____
_____
_____
_____
_____
_____
_____
_____

Month _____

	Start Fast	End Fast	Calories	Carbs	Fat	Protein	Journal?
SUNDAY							
MONDAY							
TUESDAY							
WEDNESDAY							
THURSDAY							
FRIDAY							
SATURDAY							

Month 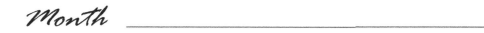 _____

SUNDAY _____

MONDAY _____

TUESDAY _____

WEDNESDAY _____

THURSDAY _____

FRIDAY _____

SATURDAY _____

GOALS/ PRIORITIES
_____
_____
_____
_____
_____
_____
_____
_____
_____
_____
_____
_____
_____

TASKS / TO DOs
_____
_____
_____
_____
_____
_____
_____
_____
_____
_____
_____
_____
_____
_____

Month _____

	Start Fast	End Fast	Calories	Carbs	Fat	Protein	Journal?
SUNDAY							
MONDAY							
TUESDAY							
WEDNESDAY							
THURSDAY							
FRIDAY							
SATURDAY							

DID I FULFILL MY INTENTIONS THIS MONTH?

___ 1. _____
___ 2. _____
___ 3. _____
___ 4. _____
___ 5. _____
___ 6. _____
___ 7. _____
___ 8. _____
___ 9. _____
___ 10. _____
___ 11. _____
___ 12. _____

What went right?

What went wrong?

LESSONS LEARNED THIS MONTH

What steps can I take to improve my results next month?

____ _____
____ _____
____ _____
____ _____
____ _____
____ _____
____ _____
____ _____
____ _____
____ _____
____ _____

Biggest lesson learned

NSVs for the month

Reward for this month

Month _____ *Year* _____

SUN	MON	TUES	WED	THURS	FRI	SAT

GOALS AND INTENTIONS FOR THE MONTH

Week 1

1. _____

2. _____

3. _____

Week 2

1. _____

2. _____

3. _____

Week 3

1. _____

2. _____

3. _____

Week 4

1. _____

2. _____

3. _____

Month 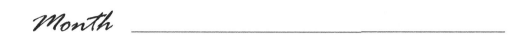 _____

SUNDAY _____

GOALS/ PRIORITIES _____

_____
_____
_____
_____

MONDAY _____

_____
_____
_____
_____
_____

TUESDAY _____

_____
_____
_____
_____
_____

WEDNESDAY _____

_____

TASKS / TO DOs _____

_____
_____
_____

THURSDAY _____

_____
_____
_____
_____

FRIDAY _____

_____
_____
_____
_____
_____

SATURDAY _____

_____
_____

_____

Month _____

	Start Fast	End Fast	Calories	Carbs	Fat	Protein	Journal?
SUNDAY							
MONDAY							
TUESDAY							
WEDNESDAY							
THURSDAY							
FRIDAY							
SATURDAY							

Month 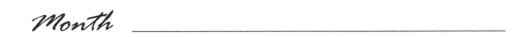 _____

SUNDAY
_____

GOALS/ PRIORITIES
_____
_____
_____
_____
_____

MONDAY
_____

_____
_____
_____
_____
_____

TUESDAY
_____

_____
_____
_____
_____
_____

WEDNESDAY
_____

_____
_____

TASKS / TO DOs
_____
_____
_____

THURSDAY
_____

_____
_____
_____
_____
_____

FRIDAY
_____

_____
_____
_____
_____
_____

SATURDAY
_____

_____
_____
_____

_____

Month _____

	Start Fast	End Fast	Calories	Carbs	Fat	Protein	Journal?
SUNDAY							
MONDAY							
TUESDAY							
WEDNESDAY							
THURSDAY							
FRIDAY							
SATURDAY							

Month 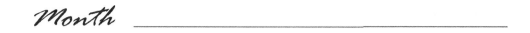 _____

SUNDAY _____

MONDAY _____

TUESDAY _____

WEDNESDAY _____

THURSDAY _____

FRIDAY _____

SATURDAY _____

GOALS/ PRIORITIES
_____
_____
_____
_____
_____
_____
_____
_____
_____
_____
_____
_____
_____
_____
_____

TASKS / TO DOs
_____
_____
_____
_____
_____
_____
_____
_____
_____
_____
_____
_____
_____
_____
_____

Month _____

	Start Fast	End Fast	Calories	Carbs	Fat	Protein	Journal?
SUNDAY							
MONDAY							
TUESDAY							
WEDNESDAY							
THURSDAY							
FRIDAY							
SATURDAY							

Month 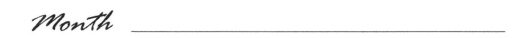 _____

SUNDAY _____

GOALS/ PRIORITIES _____
_____
_____
_____
_____
MONDAY _____
_____
_____
_____
_____
_____
_____
TUESDAY _____
_____
_____
_____
_____
_____
_____
WEDNESDAY _____
_____

TASKS / TO DOs _____
_____
_____
THURSDAY _____
_____
_____
_____
_____
_____
FRIDAY _____
_____
_____
_____
_____
_____
SATURDAY _____
_____
_____

Month _____

	Start Fast	End Fast	Calories	Carbs	Fat	Protein	Journal?
SUNDAY							
MONDAY							
TUESDAY							
WEDNESDAY							
THURSDAY							
FRIDAY							
SATURDAY							

Month 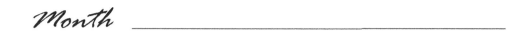 _____

SUNDAY _____

MONDAY _____

TUESDAY _____

WEDNESDAY _____

THURSDAY _____

FRIDAY _____

SATURDAY _____

GOALS/ PRIORITIES
_____
_____
_____
_____
_____
_____
_____
_____
_____
_____
_____
_____
_____
_____

TASKS / TO DOs
_____
_____
_____
_____
_____
_____
_____
_____
_____
_____
_____
_____
_____

Month _____

	Start Fast	End Fast	Calories	Carbs	Fat	Protein	Journal?
SUNDAY							
MONDAY							
TUESDAY							
WEDNESDAY							
THURSDAY							
FRIDAY							
SATURDAY							

DID I FULFILL MY INTENTIONS THIS MONTH?

___ 1. _____
___ 2. _____
___ 3. _____
___ 4. _____
___ 5. _____
___ 6. _____
___ 7. _____
___ 8. _____
___ 9. _____
___ 10. _____
___ 11. _____
___ 12. _____

What went right?

What went wrong?

LESSONS LEARNED THIS MONTH

What steps can I take to improve my results next month?

___ _____
___ _____
___ _____
___ _____
___ _____
___ _____
___ _____
___ _____
___ _____
___ _____
___ _____

Biggest lesson learned	NSVs for the month

Reward for this month

Month _____ *Year* _____

SUN	MON	TUES	WED	THURS	FRI	SAT

GOALS AND INTENTIONS FOR THE MONTH

Week 1

1. _____

2. _____

3. _____

_____

Week 2

1. _____

2. _____

3. _____

_____

Week 3

1. _____

2. _____

3. _____

_____

Week 4

1. _____

2. _____

3. _____

_____

Month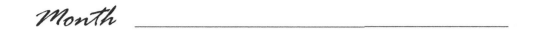

SUNDAY

MONDAY

TUESDAY

WEDNESDAY

THURSDAY

FRIDAY

SATURDAY

GOALS/ PRIORITIES

TASKS / TO DOs

Month _____

	Start Fast	End Fast	Calories	Carbs	Fat	Protein	Journal?
SUNDAY							
MONDAY							
TUESDAY							
WEDNESDAY							
THURSDAY							
FRIDAY							
SATURDAY							

Month 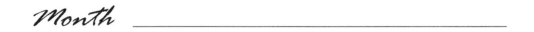 _____

SUNDAY

MONDAY

TUESDAY

WEDNESDAY

THURSDAY

FRIDAY

SATURDAY

GOALS/ PRIORITIES

TASKS / TO DOs

Month _____

	Start Fast	End Fast	Calories	Carbs	Fat	Protein	Journal?
SUNDAY							
MONDAY							
TUESDAY							
WEDNESDAY							
THURSDAY							
FRIDAY							
SATURDAY							

Month 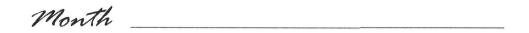 _____

SUNDAY
_____

MONDAY
_____

TUESDAY
_____

WEDNESDAY
_____

THURSDAY
_____

FRIDAY
_____

SATURDAY
_____

GOALS/ PRIORITIES
_____
_____
_____
_____
_____
_____
_____
_____
_____
_____
_____
_____
_____
_____

TASKS / TO DOs
_____
_____
_____
_____
_____
_____
_____
_____
_____
_____
_____
_____
_____
_____
_____
_____

Month _____

	Start Fast	End Fast	Calories	Carbs	Fat	Protein	Journal?
SUNDAY							
MONDAY							
TUESDAY							
WEDNESDAY							
THURSDAY							
FRIDAY							
SATURDAY							

Month 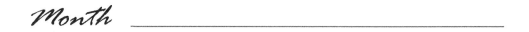 _____

SUNDAY
_____

MONDAY
_____

TUESDAY
_____

WEDNESDAY
_____

THURSDAY
_____

FRIDAY
_____

SATURDAY
_____

GOALS/ PRIORITIES
_____
_____
_____
_____
_____
_____
_____
_____
_____
_____
_____
_____
_____
_____

TASKS / TO DOs
_____
_____
_____
_____
_____
_____
_____
_____
_____
_____
_____
_____

Month _____

	Start Fast	End Fast	Calories	Carbs	Fat	Protein	Journal?
SUNDAY							
MONDAY							
TUESDAY							
WEDNESDAY							
THURSDAY							
FRIDAY							
SATURDAY							

Month 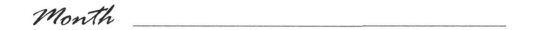 _____

SUNDAY

MONDAY

TUESDAY

WEDNESDAY

THURSDAY

FRIDAY

SATURDAY

GOALS/ PRIORITIES

TASKS / TO DOs

Month _____

	Start Fast	End Fast	Calories	Carbs	Fat	Protein	Journal?
SUNDAY							
MONDAY							
TUESDAY							
WEDNESDAY							
THURSDAY							
FRIDAY							
SATURDAY							

DID I FULFILL MY INTENTIONS THIS MONTH?

___ 1. _____

___ 2. _____

___ 3. _____

___ 4. _____

___ 5. _____

___ 6. _____

___ 7. _____

___ 8. _____

___ 9. _____

___ 10. _____

___ 11. _____

___ 12. _____

What went right?

What went wrong?

LESSONS LEARNED THIS MONTH

What steps can I take to improve my results next month?

___ _____
___ _____
___ _____
___ _____
___ _____
___ _____
___ _____
___ _____
___ _____
___ _____
___ _____
___ _____

Biggest lesson learned	NSVs for the month

Reward for this month

Month _____ *Year* _____

SUN	MON	TUES	WED	THURS	FRI	SAT

GOALS AND INTENTIONS FOR THE MONTH

Week 1

1. _____
2. _____
3. _____

Week 2

1. _____
2. _____
3. _____

Week 3

1. _____
2. _____
3. _____

Week 4

1. _____
2. _____
3. _____

Month 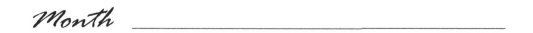 _____

SUNDAY _____

MONDAY _____

TUESDAY _____

WEDNESDAY _____

THURSDAY _____

FRIDAY _____

SATURDAY _____

GOALS/ PRIORITIES
_____
_____
_____
_____
_____
_____
_____
_____
_____
_____
_____
_____
_____

TASKS / TO DOs
_____
_____
_____
_____
_____
_____
_____
_____
_____
_____
_____
_____
_____
_____

Month _____

	Start Fast	End Fast	Calories	Carbs	Fat	Protein	Journal?
SUNDAY							
MONDAY							
TUESDAY							
WEDNESDAY							
THURSDAY							
FRIDAY							
SATURDAY							

Month 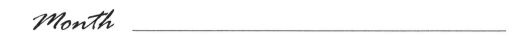 _____

SUNDAY _____

MONDAY _____

TUESDAY _____

WEDNESDAY _____

THURSDAY _____

FRIDAY _____

SATURDAY _____

GOALS/ PRIORITIES
_____
_____
_____
_____
_____
_____
_____
_____
_____
_____
_____
_____
_____
_____
_____

TASKS / TO DOs
_____
_____
_____
_____
_____
_____
_____
_____
_____
_____
_____
_____

Month _____

	Start Fast	End Fast	Calories	Carbs	Fat	Protein	Journal?
SUNDAY							
MONDAY							
TUESDAY							
WEDNESDAY							
THURSDAY							
FRIDAY							
SATURDAY							

Month 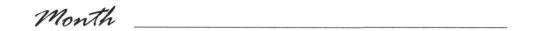 _____

SUNDAY

MONDAY

TUESDAY

WEDNESDAY

THURSDAY

FRIDAY

SATURDAY

GOALS/ PRIORITIES

TASKS / TO DOs

Month _____

	Start Fast	End Fast	Calories	Carbs	Fat	Protein	Journal?
SUNDAY							
MONDAY							
TUESDAY							
WEDNESDAY							
THURSDAY							
FRIDAY							
SATURDAY							

Month 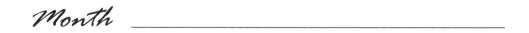 _____

SUNDAY
_____

MONDAY
_____

TUESDAY
_____

WEDNESDAY
_____

THURSDAY
_____

FRIDAY
_____

SATURDAY
_____

GOALS/ PRIORITIES
_____
_____
_____
_____
_____
_____
_____
_____
_____
_____
_____
_____
_____
_____
_____
_____

TASKS / TO DOs
_____
_____
_____
_____
_____
_____
_____
_____
_____
_____
_____
_____
_____
_____
_____

Month _____

	Start Fast	End Fast	Calories	Carbs	Fat	Protein	Journal?
SUNDAY							
MONDAY							
TUESDAY							
WEDNESDAY							
THURSDAY							
FRIDAY							
SATURDAY							

Month 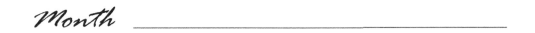 _____

SUNDAY
_____

GOALS/ PRIORITIES
_____
_____
_____
_____
_____

MONDAY
_____
_____
_____
_____
_____

TUESDAY
_____
_____
_____
_____
_____
_____

WEDNESDAY
_____
_____

TASKS / TO DOs
_____
_____
_____
_____

THURSDAY
_____
_____
_____
_____
_____

FRIDAY
_____
_____
_____
_____
_____

SATURDAY
_____
_____

Month _____

	Start Fast	End Fast	Calories	Carbs	Fat	Protein	Journal?
SUNDAY							
MONDAY							
TUESDAY							
WEDNESDAY							
THURSDAY							
FRIDAY							
SATURDAY							

DID I FULFILL MY INTENTIONS THIS MONTH?

____ 1. _____

____ 2. _____

____ 3. _____

____ 4. _____

____ 5. _____

____ 6. _____

____ 7. _____

____ 8. _____

____ 9. _____

____ 10. _____

____ 11. _____

____ 12. _____

What went right?

What went wrong?

LESSONS LEARNED THIS MONTH

What steps can I take to improve my results next month?

_____

_____

_____

_____

_____

_____

_____

_____

_____

_____

_____

_____

Biggest lesson learned	NSVs for the month

Reward for this month

Month _____ *Year* _____

SUN	MON	TUES	WED	THURS	FRI	SAT

GOALS AND INTENTIONS FOR THE MONTH

Week 1

1. _____

2. _____

3. _____

Week 2

1. _____

2. _____

3. _____

Week 3

1. _____

2. _____

3. _____

Week 4

1. _____

2. _____

3. _____

Month 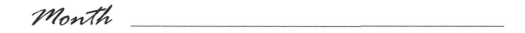 _____

SUNDAY _____

MONDAY _____

TUESDAY _____

WEDNESDAY _____

THURSDAY _____

FRIDAY _____

SATURDAY _____

GOALS/ PRIORITIES
_____
_____
_____
_____
_____
_____
_____
_____
_____
_____
_____
_____
_____

TASKS / TO DOs
_____
_____
_____
_____
_____
_____
_____
_____
_____
_____
_____
_____
_____
_____

Month _____

	Start Fast	End Fast	Calories	Carbs	Fat	Protein	Journal?
SUNDAY							
MONDAY							
TUESDAY							
WEDNESDAY							
THURSDAY							
FRIDAY							
SATURDAY							

Month 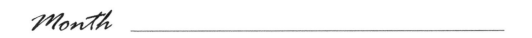 _____

SUNDAY

GOALS/ PRIORITIES

MONDAY

TUESDAY

WEDNESDAY

TASKS / TO DOs

THURSDAY

FRIDAY

SATURDAY

Month _____

	Start Fast	End Fast	Calories	Carbs	Fat	Protein	Journal?
SUNDAY							
MONDAY							
TUESDAY							
WEDNESDAY							
THURSDAY							
FRIDAY							
SATURDAY							

Month 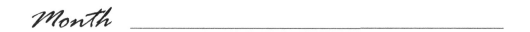 _____

SUNDAY _____

GOALS/ PRIORITIES

_____
_____
_____
_____
_____

MONDAY _____

_____
_____
_____
_____
_____

TUESDAY _____

_____
_____
_____
_____
_____

WEDNESDAY _____

_____
_____

TASKS / TO DOs

_____
_____
_____

THURSDAY _____

_____
_____
_____
_____
_____

FRIDAY _____

_____
_____
_____
_____

SATURDAY _____

_____
_____
_____

Month _____

	Start Fast	End Fast	Calories	Carbs	Fat	Protein	Journal?
SUNDAY							
MONDAY							
TUESDAY							
WEDNESDAY							
THURSDAY							
FRIDAY							
SATURDAY							

Month 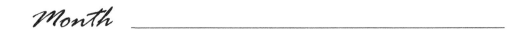 _____

SUNDAY _____

GOALS/ PRIORITIES
_____
_____
_____
_____

MONDAY _____

_____
_____
_____
_____

TUESDAY _____

_____
_____
_____
_____

WEDNESDAY _____

_____
_____

TASKS / TO DOs
_____

THURSDAY _____

_____
_____
_____
_____

FRIDAY _____

_____
_____
_____
_____

SATURDAY _____

_____
_____
_____

Month _____

	Start Fast	End Fast	Calories	Carbs	Fat	Protein	Journal?
SUNDAY							
MONDAY							
TUESDAY							
WEDNESDAY							
THURSDAY							
FRIDAY							
SATURDAY							

Month 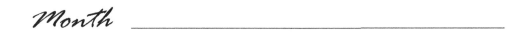 _____

SUNDAY

GOALS/ PRIORITIES

MONDAY

TUESDAY

WEDNESDAY

TASKS / TO DOs

THURSDAY

FRIDAY

SATURDAY

Month _____

	Start Fast	End Fast	Calories	Carbs	Fat	Protein	Journal?
SUNDAY							
MONDAY							
TUESDAY							
WEDNESDAY							
THURSDAY							
FRIDAY							
SATURDAY							

DID I FULFILL MY INTENTIONS THIS MONTH?

____ 1. _____
____ 2. _____
____ 3. _____
____ 4. _____
____ 5. _____
____ 6. _____
____ 7. _____
____ 8. _____
____ 9. _____
____ 10. _____
____ 11. _____
____ 12. _____

What went right?

What went wrong?

LESSONS LEARNED THIS MONTH

What steps can I take to improve my results next month?

_____ _____

_____ _____

_____ _____

_____ _____

_____ _____

_____ _____

_____ _____

_____ _____

_____ _____

_____ _____

_____ _____

Biggest lesson learned

NSVs for the month

Reward for this month

Month _____ *Year* _____

SUN	MON	TUES	WED	THURS	FRI	SAT

GOALS AND INTENTIONS FOR THE MONTH

Week 1

1. _____
2. _____
3. _____
_____

Week 2

1. _____
2. _____
3. _____
_____

Week 3

1. _____
2. _____
3. _____
_____

Week 4

1. _____
2. _____
3. _____
_____

Month 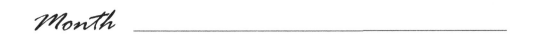 _____

SUNDAY _____

GOALS/ PRIORITIES

_____
_____
_____
_____

MONDAY _____

_____
_____
_____
_____

TUESDAY _____

_____
_____
_____
_____

WEDNESDAY _____

_____

TASKS / TO DOs

_____
_____
_____
_____

THURSDAY _____

_____
_____
_____
_____

FRIDAY _____

_____
_____
_____
_____

SATURDAY _____

_____

Month _____

	Start Fast	End Fast	Calories	Carbs	Fat	Protein	Journal?
SUNDAY							
MONDAY							
TUESDAY							
WEDNESDAY							
THURSDAY							
FRIDAY							
SATURDAY							

Month 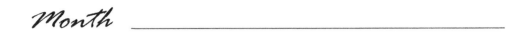 _____

SUNDAY	GOALS/ PRIORITIES
MONDAY	
TUESDAY	
WEDNESDAY	
	TASKS / TO DOs
THURSDAY	
FRIDAY	
SATURDAY	

Month _____

	Start Fast	End Fast	Calories	Carbs	Fat	Protein	Journal?
SUNDAY							
MONDAY							
TUESDAY							
WEDNESDAY							
THURSDAY							
FRIDAY							
SATURDAY							

Month 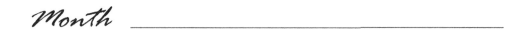 _____

SUNDAY _____

MONDAY _____

TUESDAY _____

WEDNESDAY _____

THURSDAY _____

FRIDAY _____

SATURDAY _____

GOALS/ PRIORITIES
_____
_____
_____
_____
_____
_____
_____
_____
_____
_____
_____
_____
_____
_____

TASKS / TO DOs
_____
_____
_____
_____
_____
_____
_____
_____
_____
_____
_____
_____
_____
_____

Month _____

	Start Fast	End Fast	Calories	Carbs	Fat	Protein	Journal?
SUNDAY							
MONDAY							
TUESDAY							
WEDNESDAY							
THURSDAY							
FRIDAY							
SATURDAY							

Month 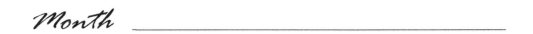 _____

SUNDAY
_____

GOALS/ PRIORITIES
_____
_____
_____
_____

MONDAY
_____
_____
_____
_____
_____

TUESDAY
_____
_____
_____
_____
_____
_____

WEDNESDAY
_____
_____

TASKS / TO DOs
_____
_____
_____

THURSDAY
_____
_____
_____
_____

FRIDAY
_____
_____
_____
_____

SATURDAY
_____

_____

Month _____

	Start Fast	End Fast	Calories	Carbs	Fat	Protein	Journal?
SUNDAY							
MONDAY							
TUESDAY							
WEDNESDAY							
THURSDAY							
FRIDAY							
SATURDAY							

Month 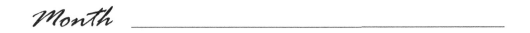 _____

SUNDAY
_____

MONDAY
_____

TUESDAY
_____

WEDNESDAY
_____

THURSDAY
_____

FRIDAY
_____

SATURDAY
_____

GOALS/ PRIORITIES
_____
_____
_____
_____
_____
_____
_____
_____
_____
_____
_____
_____
_____
_____
_____

TASKS / TO DOs
_____
_____
_____
_____
_____
_____
_____
_____
_____
_____
_____
_____
_____
_____
_____
_____

Month _____

	Start Fast	End Fast	Calories	Carbs	Fat	Protein	Journal?
SUNDAY							
MONDAY							
TUESDAY							
WEDNESDAY							
THURSDAY							
FRIDAY							
SATURDAY							

DID I FULFILL MY INTENTIONS THIS MONTH?

___ 1. _____
___ 2. _____
___ 3. _____
___ 4. _____
___ 5. _____
___ 6. _____
___ 7. _____
___ 8. _____
___ 9. _____
___ 10. _____
___ 11. _____
___ 12. _____

What went right?

What went wrong?

LESSONS LEARNED THIS MONTH

What steps can I take to improve my results next month?

___ _____
___ _____
___ _____
___ _____
___ _____
___ _____
___ _____
___ _____
___ _____
___ _____
___ _____
___ _____

Biggest lesson learned

NSVs for the month

Reward for this month

If you found this book useful,
please leave a review.
Thank you!

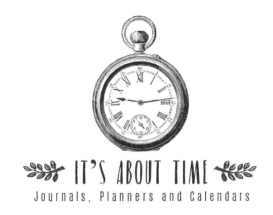

IT'S ABOUT TIME
Journals, Planners and Calendars

Contact us: Info@ItsAboutTimeBooks.com

© 2019 ItsAboutTimeBooks.com.
All rights reserved.

*No part of this publication may be reproduced, replicated,
redistributed or given away in any form without the prior
written consent of the author/publisher or the terms
conveyed herein to the purchaser.*

Made in the USA
Monee, IL
08 April 2022

94377483R00063